50 Things to Know

50 THINGS TO KNOW ABOUT BEING A RIDESHARE OR DELIVERY DRIVER

A DRIVER GUIDEBOOK

SILVAIN ALARILLA

50 Things to Know Being a Rideshare and Delivery Driver Copyright © 2019 by CZYK Publishing LLC. All Rights Reserved.

All rights reserved. No part of this book may be reproduced in any form or by any electronic or mechanical means including information storage and retrieval systems, without permission in writing from the author. The only exception is by a reviewer, who may quote short excerpts in a review.

The statements in this book are of the authors and may not be the views of CZYK Publishing or 50 Things to Know.

Cover designed by: Ivana Stamenkovic
Cover Image: https://pixabay.com/photos/car-traffic-man-hurry-1149997/

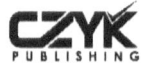

CZYK Publishing Since 2011.

50 Things to Know
Visit our website at 50thingstoknow.com

Lock Haven, PA
All rights reserved.
ISBN: 9781091869448

50 THINGS TO KNOW ABOUT BEING A RIDESHARE AND DELIVERY DRIVER

BOOK DESCRIPTION

Do you want to supplement your income?

Do you want to have a flexible schedule?

Do you want to start working on your own terms?

If you answered yes to any of these questions then this book is for you...

50 Things to Know About Being a Rideshare and Delivery Driver by Silvain Alarilla offers an approach to learning how to earn through rideshare and delivery apps in a fun way. Most of the information about using rideshare and delivery apps can be found in blog or subreddits. Although there's nothing wrong with looking for information there, this book compiles all that, in addition to my tips based on my real-life experiences from using multiple apps.

In these pages you'll discover what you need to know before you start trying any of the rideshare apps. This book will help you set expectations and lessen your anxiety about trying something new.

By the time you finish this book, you will know how to make your rideshare experience fun and hopefully profitable. So grab YOUR copy today. You'll be glad you did.

TABLE OF CONTENTS

50 Things to Know
Book Series
Reviews from Readers
Silvain Alarilla
BOOK DESCRIPTION
TABLE OF CONTENTS
DEDICATION
ABOUT THE AUTHOR
INTRODUCTION
1. Mind Your Business
2. You're Not In A Race
3. Doing Uber
4. Delivering For Uber Eats
5. Giving Lyfts
6. Doordashing
7. Grubhubbing
8. Postmates
9. Caviar
10. Check Your City's Requirement
11. Do Your Own Taxes
12. Call Your Car Insurance
13. Heads up: There's no 401k
14. Getting Gas?
15. Get A Carwash Membership

16. Be The Friendly Local
17. Check What's Under Your Hood
18. Think Of Where You Are Driving
19. Dress To (Sort Of) Impress
20. Treat Your Guests
21. Watch Your Smell
22. Be Like Aoki
23. Keep it PG
24. Keep It Fresh
25. Keep Your Personal Data To Yourself
26. Your Ratings Is How They Watch You
27. Do Not Wander Aimlessly
28. Mind Your Bladder
29. Driving In The 'Burbs
30. When Doing Airport Pick-ups and Drop-offs
31. Picking-up From the Land and Sea
32. Be A Team Player
33. Give That Party Animal A Ride
34. Give Service Animals a Lift Too
35. Park It While It's Hot
36. Getting Food On The Go
37. Bring Water
38. Going On A Quest
39. Keep it Handy
40. Check For Spoils
41. Keep Updated

42. Get Matching Trips
43. Roadtripping
44. Doing Car Pools
45. Make Conversation
46. Talk To Other Drivers
47. Rate Your Riders and Deliveries
48. Don't Get Deactivated
49. You Got To Hustle Hard
50. Be Fun! Have Fun!

Other Helpful Resources

50 Things to Know

DEDICATION

This is for anyone who needs a fresh start. To anyone who needs a break from the madness.

ABOUT THE AUTHOR

Silvain Alarilla may not be a household name or a known source of infinite wisdom but he has been busy living life and documenting what he sees, hears, and feels. He is a writer after all, among other things. He started to rideshare during the summer of 2019 while working on his first book. He felt like he needed to quit his last job but still needed something to pay the bills. He has collected the things he has learned in this book, in hopes that it can help others who have no idea on how to start the hustle.

He is currently working on remodeling his blogs and will hopefully rerelease "Snor's Kitchen" in 2019. You can find out more about him and his blogs on his Amazon author page:

amazon.com/author/silvainalarilla

You can connect with him on twitter:

twitter.com/slvnanthny

INTRODUCTION

"Nothing behind me, everything ahead of me, as is ever so on the road. "

- On the Road, Jack Kerouac

It just hit me one day. I was earning money through an app. I was following the commands and prompts of the machine and I get compensated well if I do a good job. You go wherever the app takes you. Before cars learn how to drive for themselves, they have us.

It may seem like a simple enough job for some. For some, it is pretty much, just driving around right? You can over simplify it to just that and overlook how much you have to hustle hard to profit. Don't worry. There will be always something better. If it isn't this gig or that job. It doesn't matter. All that matters, is that you keep moving.

As of 2018, roughly a third of the workers in the U.S. are participating in the gig economy. What is the gig worker? They are independent contractors that earn through means outside of the traditional long-term work. The great thing about it is that it might take only a few days before you can start working. It honestly beats staying at home, hoping for money to rain.

1. MIND YOUR BUSINESS

When you drive for rideshares on a full-time basis, who do you think you have to answer to? The answer is yourself. You're the one who decides whether you wake up early for the morning rush or brave the stress of the evening rush hour. On the flip-side, you also decide if you want to do nothing and take some hopefully well deserved, time-off. Your time is your greatest asset. You're also providing a service that gives convenience to your consumer. Your customers can choose to walk, take the bus, hop on the train, or just stay at home and save their money. Your responsibility is to bring someone or their food from point A to point B in the safest, most timely, and most convenient way possible. Time is also your product. It is the time you save the clients. Remember the value that you give and let your business or side gig grow.

2. YOU'RE NOT IN A RACE

Although it is important to be on time when serving your clients, you don't have to play catch-up by speeding. If you find yourself late, just try to look forward and focus on what time you can save. It will not save you time if you get pulled over for speeding. If you think about it more and contemplate the basic economics of it, when you drive sensibly, you can save yourself the tire wear, save on gas consumption, and prevent the stress of sudden braking on your brake pads. You can also get better tips from passengers if you don't drive like a maniac.

3. DOING UBER

Inventions and innovation are bred from inconvenience. This was the case for the founders of Uber, Travis Kalanick and Garret Camp, who had trouble catching a cab on a December evening in Paris (2008). They then launched their game changing app, Uber a year after in San Francisco, California. This was also the first driving app that I tried. In my opinion, the Uber driver app is the easiest to use. It's the most handsfree app in the sense that I don't get as distracted by having to tap on my app during pick-ups and drop offs frequently like in the Lyft app. The app is easy to start as well as navigate around in. Signing up is easy as well. It only took me couple of days to be able to start.

The first step was booking an appointment at my nearest Uber Greenlight location. There I did a test on how much I knew the Seattle Metro Area. I filled out some forms and had a vehicle inspection. It might even be easier to start in other places. The ease and convenience does come at a price: Uber takes 25% from the rides you do. The purpose of this fee is for the use of the Uber driver app, the collection and transfer of fares, credit card commission, and distribution of invoices to clients.

4. DELIVERING FOR UBER EATS

Once you get the hang of the Uber app, you may want to consider doing food deliveries. Food deliveries don't pay as much, and sometimes it requires more work, but it keeps the time filled. The busiest times for meals are during lunch and dinner. I used to get a lot of breakfast requests before I reach downtown Seattle when I drove in the morning. Before you start you must buy thermal bags unless Uber provides you with one. I didn't get one when I started. Make sure you get good and sturdy ones. The ones I got from the dollar store didn't work out so well. The ability to delivery your food at the desired temperature can contribute on how much of tip you will get. Having at least two bags, a cold one and a hot one, is the key to keeping the right serving temperature. It can also be helpful to have a designated drink container to prevent spills. It is easy to find in Amazon or at your local retail store.

5. GIVING LYFTS

Who would we be without our competitors? Lyft is another rideshare company based in San Francisco. The Uber competitor started in 2012 and is a current competitor in the Seattle Metro Area. I tried using the Lyft app a month after trying Uber. I would switch from one app to the other if the driver demand was low. I personally had more calls for rides using Uber but it seems like Lyft pays better. Apparently Lyft actually does pay better, and charges only 20% plus the full booking fee.

In my experience, Uber has the better and simpler app. Pick-ups can be confusing since the GPS can lead you to an apartment or commercial building as a pick-up point but you actually have to follow the client icon with their actual location.

6. DOORDASHING

The app's name is accurate to what you essentially do. Run that delivery to your client's door. Unfortunately, Doordash can fail to provide their drivers an adequate time to complete deliveries. It was tested on the first time I tried Doordash. It was almost comedic how much my greed took over and was immediately enticed by a $5 bonus per delivery without question. Unknown to me was a Cheescake Factory and Doordash promo. Everybody's father, mother, brother, and sister ordered something from Cheesecake Factory and had their free cheesecake or whatever the freebie was. There was barely any parking but I was lucky to catch another dasher leaving their spot. I was greeted by other dashers wishing me luck.

I was again welcomed by a line that started from the cheesecake takeout section, curving up before it reached the restroom, and continued the line in the hallway between a few customers having lunch. We were standing awkwardly holding the free red Doordash insulated bag. I felt like a huge wall blocking the servers from their tables and making people hungry. The time in line gave me a chance to study the app. It switches from the Doordash app to Google maps when you start navigating. A way to go around this is using multiple app setting on your phone if it can do so. It also reminded me of checking if I carried my "redcard" to pay for orders that still require payments or actual ordering. In Cheesecake Factory's case, they prepack the meals to fit inside the insulated bags. Sometimes their packaging can be large though. When I picked up the order, I was already late for my delivery. When I got to the apartment I was delivering at, the customer neglected to place their apartment number. Luckily, I was able to contact them by phone and finally made my drop-off.

Fortunately, epic deliveries like that aren't the norm (I guess). An advantage of using Doordash is that you can choose which area you want to work on. I worked Doordash mostly in the suburbs, like Renton and Tukwila, sometimes South Seattle. It was helpful that I was able to familiarize myself with a specific area only. It makes deliveries much more efficient but only to a point. You can schedule your dash ahead of time or choose to "dash now" in the areas needed. When it gets busier, Doordash offers "bonuses" per delivery. Usually it's just a dollar or two. You can get the bonus on completed deliveries during the bonus period as long as you have the acceptance rate of 80%.

Although clients can tip the drivers, I don't know if Doordash makes it that well known to customers. I rarely made tips with Doordash. Even when I did everything right and on time. I even had a customer order $80 worth of food, have a far delivery distance, and then tip 50 cents. It can be disheartening since Doordash has a flat base rate for deliveries, even if the delivery location is 20 minutes away. It was like earning less than minimum wage at times.

7. GRUBHUBBING

One day, while I was doing ride for Uber, I was able to talk my rider about Doordash being my other side hustle. He adamantly said, "Don't do Doordash." He mentioned that he had been doing deliveries only and has been doing Grubhub and Postmates. He said that Grubhub pays more and customers tend to tip better. He continued to say that he would go online on Postmates after his scheduled block on Grubhub. The conversation had to end when I dropped him off but that's when I started comparing all the delivery services.

Grubhub pays for your time and the distance you travelled from where you pick-up. They also claim that you receive %100 of your tips. I did notice that Grubhub paid the most per delivery but you had to go closer to center of the metro area you are assigned to, to be able to get more delivery requests. You can also set-up a "block", ahead of time when you are notified by the app of their availability. I did notice that their blocks tend to get full quickly, compared to other delivery apps. Blocks come in hour increments, think of it like a short, assigned shift. If available, I try to start a block as early as 11am for the lunch rush and 4pm for the dinner rush. The great thing about Grubhub is that they guarantee you $15 for each block assigned to you ahead of time. If you didn't get any requests during your 1-hour block, you would still get $15 from them. You must complete all orders, as well as receive all requests, to get the guaranteed rate. Grubhub also provides their riders with a huge insulated bag for pizza aside from the regular sized insulated bag.

8. POSTMATES

I honestly preferred this app the least, but it can still be useful when you find yourself without any customers. Driving for Postmates can kind of feel like being someone's personal shopper. Their kit comes with a bag and debit card to be used for payments on deliveries. With Postmates, you would have to take a few more steps because instead of just picking up an order; you must fall in line, make the order, pay for it using the assigned debit card, take a picture of the receipt using the app, and then pick up the order. It may not seem like that much extra work, but you might find yourself spending more time than you want on an order which won't pay much upfront. Another con for using Postmates is that your tip payments are also delayed at times. It makes it harder to keep track of how much you are really making. Although I would not start my day with going online with Postmates, I still like getting that little extra deposit from them from time to time.

9. CAVIAR

This food delivery company was acquired by Square, Inc. which provides small businesses the capability to make mobile payments. Prior to being bought, Caviar only provided customers with the service of being able to order food online for pick-up. Square expanded the business by allowing food deliveries.

With Caviar, you have to provide your own insulated bag for regular deliveries and pizza. You must submit photographic proof via email before you can start. You can get this from Caviar's online store but you are also free to buy other brands. I even used my Grubhub bag instead of buying a new one. It might just be confusing for some vendors when you come in. Upon signing up, I was also prompted to download and use the Cash app for direct deposits. The app was also developed by Square, Inc and can be used as a digital wallet. Aside from US dollars, you can buy, sell and hold Bitcoin. Although this app is optional when using Caviar, I still like using it to keep my extra earnings from Caviar, as well as buying crypto.

Caviar's delivery app is also easy to use and is similar to the Uber app except it does not have its own navigation in the app. For the Seattle Metro Area, it seemed like Caviar was busier closer to downtown, unlike Uber Eats and Doordash, which had frequent requests in the suburbs of the Seattle Metro Area. Caviar customers also seem to tip better than the ones using Doordash in my experience. Deposits are also easily made when I used the Cash App.

10. CHECK YOUR CITY'S REQUIREMENT

Remember regular taxi cabs? They are licensed and inspected by the city, and maybe even paying more than what Uber or Lyft drivers pay to start. With the free market and privatization, it is only natural that Uber was able to cut corners and run with less regulation. But as cities continue to have more demand for rideshare services, the more the cities try to regulate. Check your city requirements or face penalties or deactivation.

For the city of Seattle, drivers you must acquire a TNC (Transportation Network Companies) rideshare permit, a city business license, as well as a for-hire driver's license. You also must make sure that what you are driving is up to date. When I started last year in 2018, Uber was only allowing cars made from 2013 or newer.

11. DO YOUR OWN TAXES

I would suggest talking to a tax expert if taxes go over your head. When you earn more than $600 in your small business, the rideshare or delivery company will send you a 1099 form. Remember that your rides haven't been taxed yet. Keep that in mind whenever you get your earnings, make sure that you set a certain amount aside for taxes later.

12. CALL YOUR CAR INSURANCE

Are you worried about the implications to your insurance when using your vehicle for rideshare? Make sure that your car insurance company is aware that you started ridesharing or else you may not get compensated properly in case of an accident. Doing the right thing comes with the price of an increased rate, but this is something you can expect from any car insurance company, since you have more liability now.

It is also good to know that Uber also has their car insurance when you go online. You can apply for it and cover you and your passenger when an accident occurs. It is only supplementary and that you are still required to have your own coverage.

13. HEADS UP: THERE'S NO 401K

Since it is your own small business, you cannot rely on anyone but yourself to set-up your own retirement or investment fund. Although I am not a financial advisor, I know that setting aside for the future is a must. Since the rideshare and delivery apps don't intentionally hire drivers full-time, they also don't provide a 401k. Thankfully in the age of smartphones there are apps you download to set-up your own retirement fund.

Acorns is an app that will help you invest with low maintenance required. It currently offers a core investment account for $1/month, and if you go up to $2/month you will have the Acorns Later account which has an IRA for long-term investments. You can adjust whether you want to be aggressive or conservative with the funds you own. They also provide informational resources for you to become a better investor.

An Uber suggested app is the Stash app. The apps is similar to Acorns, and has a similar rate. The advantage with Stash is that you can buy specific partial stocks from companies like Netflix and Facebook. You can also buy in terms of portfolios or group of stocks. It is similar where in you can adjust whether you are conservative or aggressive in your investments, but different wherein you get to choose the portfolio. You can even buy stocks on ETF's like Corporate Cannabis. You can purchase different portfolios on bonds.

14. GETTING GAS?

If you are used to not watching for gas prices, it is time to keep track. It's simple enough, the cheaper the gas, the better the profits. You can save up by joining a wholesale membership like Costco and also earn cashback on their executive membership. If you opened an account with GoBank when you signed-up for Uber, you can earn more cashback on gas. You can also get discounted gas prices when you frequent groceries that have gas stations.

15. GET A CARWASH MEMBERSHIP

One of the things that Uber and Lyft emphasizes is that you must have a clean car. For a fulltime rideshare/delivery driver, going to the carwash may be a daily or almost daily ritual. I bought a carwash monthly membership to bring the cost down. I go to Brown Bear to get my car washed and got the medium tier wash. Supposedly they use "eco-friendly detergents." When you reach 5 carwashes in a month, then you got your money's worth. However, I would still suggest, being mindful when going to the carwash and check if it is really needed.

16. BE THE FRIENDLY LOCAL

Being familiar with the local spots is useful especially when someone is from out of town. Giving passengers a mini-tour guide experience can get you tips, granted you also watch the road.

The same goes with being friendly with business owners and employees during deliveries. Pick-ups become easier and more fun when the locals know you. Give your friendliest smile. Don't be afraid to say hi and make some small talk. The more you know how the business operates on a food delivery level, the better the synchronicity. It's the simple things like whether or not you have to grab utensils for yourself or if they already placed it inside the sealed meal.

17. CHECK WHAT'S UNDER YOUR HOOD

It is not enough that your car made the minimum year required to drive. You must still check if everything is in working condition, even when your car is only slightly used. That tape over the check engine light is no longer a useful remedy. I had to personally spend $1500. A huge chunk of it was spent on my swapping all my tires since it was time. The rest was spent on A/C repair and regular maintenance. The repairs and maintenance for your car will dramatically increase if you drive for Uber full-time. You would have to expect that the change oil light will pop-up more since you are also driving more. To ensure that you keep on moving, be on top of your repairs and maintenance.

18. THINK OF WHERE YOU ARE DRIVING

The weather patterns in your area can affect your business. You are technically working outside after all. Stay tuned to local weather updates. You can easily install weather widgets on your phone.

If you are like me and you live somewhere that rains a lot, you might want to consider using tires that do well in wet conditions. Make sure that your wipers are also in good shape. Passengers may become weary when you are driving with lots of streaks and less visibility. Although the rain can also bring business since more people would rather call an Uber than walk under the rain, it may be more enjoyable and safer to drive under the sun, but it doesn't always mean lots of business.

Driving in the snow is my weakness and I avoid driving when it does. I moved to Seattle, thinking that it wasn't going to be too snowy, with snow only happening once or twice a year. Unfortunately, I didn't know that this city practically shuts down when it does snow. Because of all the slopes and hills in the area, it can be difficult and even dangerous to drive in the streets of Seattle. If you haven't seen the videos of cars and buses slipping around and sliding down the streets here, then doing a quick search can give you a frame of reference. During this winter's last snow storm, I just let my car hang out at our apartment's parking lot for a week. If I didn't have a full-time job at the time, I would have taken a huge loss on earnings.

It can be a problem when the heat becomes too much as well. Make sure you regularly check your car's engine temperature to prevent stoppage from overheating. Before starting, I also had to take my car in for air-conditioning repairs which caused me more than $200. The a/c might not be a big deal for some but I didn't want to give my passenger a hand fan and risk getting a 1-star rating.

19. DRESS TO (SORT OF) IMPRESS

An advantage of not having a boss, is not having a restrictive dress code. I had some days where I just wore faded sweat pants and the shirt I had on from the night before. But really in this case, your clients become your boss. Wearing something lousy and raggedy can be comfortable or easy but it will not get you tips. If you dress like you care about your job, then it may reflect on the minds of your clients.

On the flip side, make sure that you are also comfortable with what you are wearing. Remember that aside from sitting and driving for an extensive period of time, you may have to jump out of the car for deliveries or help with luggage. I like to dress as comfy as I can when I am doing deliveries just in case I have to run or walk faster. If the delivery service you are working for has a shirt or uniform, wear your swag to represent. Some establishments have more than one delivery service used so it becomes less confusing when you have an official uniform on (even if it isn't required).

20. TREAT YOUR GUESTS

People love freebies. People also like to chew on stuff when waiting. Although buying treats would have to come from your own pocket, having treats can put a smile to your riders and potentially end up in a good tip or rating especially for that sweet tooth rider of yours. Make sure you have your treats visible and offer it when you can. Aside from sweets, having mints is especially helpful for that person coming in from a restaurant or going somewhere for a date.

Having some bottled water can be helpful as well, I offer them to riders with a longer ride and/or coming from a watering hole. You can help your tipsy rider out by hydrating them.

21. WATCH YOUR SMELL

Maybe you've been there before, riding in a strange car and wondering "what's that smell?" You find yourself wondering if it is what you stepped on, sat in, or sat next to. Odors become more apparent in smaller, confined spaces. Try to avoid wearing strong scents or perfumes even if it smells good to you. The definition of what smells good can be very subjective so try to keep it neutral. I also avoid strong air fresheners as well.

Make sure you vacuum your seat covers and floor mats to avoid bits of food that may have fallen from you or the passenger and leave bad odors. The scent of smoke can linger in your car especially cigarette smoke. On the days you plan to drive, try to avoid lighting a cigarette in the car and also leave that hotbox session for another day.

22. BE LIKE AOKI

I remember when I was in college in the Philippines and used to ride these loud and colorful jeepneys down a mountain road to get home from a long day of learning about community health. They had their own playlist and blasted their music for their rider's enjoyment. It used to give me a second wind and would distract me from the crazy Metro Manila traffic. The drivers were our DJ's to the Manila Sound.

One of my goals is to provide an entertaining playlist for the commuters. I find great satisfaction when my riders start nodding their heads and singing to my tunes. It is also a great way to get a good rating. Since my playlists not only have myself in mind but also my riders, I try to play songs that are more neutral and unoffensive since you never know who's going to ride with you next. I save the songs with explicit lyrics at home or when I'm alone doing deliveries. Maybe spare some change for Ad-free streaming services like Spotify or Youtube.

23. KEEP IT PG

You have to wash your sailor's mouth with soap and water when you start doing rides. It is even part of the protocol of Uber to refrain from swearing and I would assume saying anything inappropriate would fall in the same category. It may seem like common sense to some but there are reasons for HR mediations. Be your own HR and watch yourself before you wreck yourself. If you find yourself questioning if something is appropriate to say, then maybe it really isn't.

24. KEEP IT FRESH

When doing food deliveries, you must keep the temperature right. Who likes cold pizza? Melted milkshakes? Almost no one. Before you get too excited and run off doing deliveries, make sure you have an insulated bag. You can make or break your tip when you forget your bag. Some food establishments may even reject you if you don't have one during pick-up. If you want to step up your game during deliveries, you can also use cooler gels to keeps drinks cold.

If you are delivering fries, you might have to let your insulated bag open slightly, in attempts to maintain as much of its crispiness. Be extra careful driving when delivering drinks. Sudden braking and sharp turns can end up in spills. Driving like a racer will not help either. You are not Takumi from Initial D. You will spill the tofu. Sorry for the obscure reference.

25. KEEP YOUR PERSONAL DATA TO YOURSELF

One of the first horror stories I heard from a fellow Uber driver was when someone stole his earnings. He got a call from someone posing as customer service from Uber during one his rides. He got tricked into sharing his information by accident because it sounded all too urgent. Rideshare and delivery apps typically mask your phone number from customers to prevent your data from being breached. Do not share your log-in or financial information all too readily. It is better to check your emails and confirm.

It seems like something that happens all too often since it is a common warning in the Caviar newsletter. In my case, I was delivering for Postmates. My "client" ordered just one order of small French fries from Jack-in-the-Box. I was already suspicious at the time and grew even more suspicious when I realized my delivery was addressed to a closed down store. I called my client just in case, and the person on the other end said that client cancelled their order. I checked my app and my order was still ongoing. The person on the other line posed as Postmates personnel and said that I could get an extra $10 for my delivery if I stay in the line and answer some questions. So I hung up the phone, cancelled the delivery through the app and ate my consolation fries.

26. YOUR RATINGS IS HOW THEY WATCH YOU

It's important to have a good reputation in the streets. Mind your passenger ratings as well as your acceptance and cancellation rate. Not having a direct supervisor might tempt some to slack off or go below standards, but the rating is there as an attempt to measure driver performance objectively. Better ratings mean being matched with passengers with similar ratings. Getting better ratings can also help you go up tiers. For example, Uber has their Uber Pro Partner Program. You start as a Partner, earn enough points by doing rides, then go to Gold, then Platinum, then lastly Diamond. The perks for Gold and above, start with Quest Promotions, where you earn more with consecutive rides, but more on that later. You get boosted cashback rating from 1.5% to 3%, if you use your GoBank card. If you wanted to expand your knowledge, you can also start online classes at Arizona State University for free. A great perk that starts with Gold is that you can view how far and where your next trip is. If you're worried about your car breaking down in between all your driving, you can also avail of the 24/7 roadside assistance for free! Lastly you get bragging rights and recognition through the app that you got the Gold or better. Better perks come with higher levels obviously.

27. DO NOT WANDER AIMLESSLY

Time is money, and money is gas when it comes to driving for rideshare and delivery. Remember that idling not only costs you money, but it can also have compounded effects on the environment. When I find myself in a spot with low demand, I use the app to direct me where it would most likely have more. When I find myself just driving without a passenger or delivery, I try to look for a parking spot so I can stop my engine and regroup. I open up other apps to check for demand. I also check my map if I am close to places that usually has commuters, like schools, malls or train stations. When I'm just delivering, I park by a strip mall that is close to several restaurants that offer delivery.

28. MIND YOUR BLADDER

Not everybody thinks about this, but you may encounter a difficult bathroom situation when you're ridesharing or delivering. Holding your pee may not seem like it could be dangerous but if you hold it in for too long, you may develop a Urinary Tract Infection from the bacteria hanging out and replicating in your bladder. It would be more of a bad idea if you hold your urine for long period of time when you have an enlarged prostate, neurogenic bladder, a kidney disorder, urinary retention, and a current UTI.

To avoid getting caught with public urination, I try to remember the public restrooms, fast food chains, and coffee shops in the area. It would be more courteous if you were to purchase a small item or drink when you use the restroom of a fast food chain or coffee shop. A great way to avoid that expense is to turn on your delivery app and use the restroom in your pick-up location.

29. DRIVING IN THE 'BURBS

Whenever I feel the dread of driving downtown, I contemplate on whether I should drive in the suburbs but risk the lack of demand. I end up reminding myself of the pros of staying in the 'burbs. Since it is a lot less busy, there is also a lot less traffic which can help with your gas mileage. The streets tend be less bumpy with less traffic which can prevent wear and tear from potholes and speed bumps. It's also easy to spot a public restroom when you're in a suburb that has a huge mall. The mall is also a great place to hang-out and wait for new requests. If you find yourself in the 'burbs around 3pm without a ride, head to the school and possibly pick up parents picking up their kids from school. Officially you are not allowed to have only minors in your car but I heard others experience otherwise.

30. WHEN DOING AIRPORT PICK-UPS AND DROP-OFFS

Like I said before, check your city requirements. In the Seattle-Tacoma International Airport, you are required to have a TNC permit and have a laminated blown up copy of your for-hire permit posted up front, on the passenger side of the dashboard. There are also specific places where you can pick up passengers. In Sea-Tac it's next to the Taxi queue. When dropping off at Sea-Tac early in the morning, you are supposed to drop passengers off at Arrivals instead of Departures.

These rules can change, so it is best to keep updated. If you don't follow these rules and a cop catches you, you can get fined and ticketed. If an Uber personnel catches you without the requirements, you can risk getting deactivated as well.

31. PICKING-UP FROM THE LAND AND SEA

Aside from the main airports, there are other places that require cabs to connect them to specific places. Fortunately for me, there is a Light Rail Station with a Park & Ride next to our apartment, so I usually park there first to check if there are any rider requests. They tend to be shorter rides since it's usually just someone who lives close but doesn't have a bus connection or is not willing to walk.

If your city has ferries or water taxis, take advantage and check their schedules. Not everybody who rides the ferry brings their car, so I noticed a short surge in demand when the ferry drops by. Although there aren't specific rules for picking up and dropping off at Ferry Docks, water taxis, or train stations, you must not obstruct traffic, just like everywhere else.

32. BE A TEAM PLAYER

If you really want to be someone's MVP, keep track of the games in your city and give a ride to fan. Uber usually notifies drivers when there is a big game ahead of time, so you can plan on driving. Although the light rail is available close to the stadium here in Seattle, it is still very common for people to call on an Uber or Lyft. If you can't find a ride, or the queue is too long at the stadium, you can probably find rides after the game at the watering holes nearby. Show your team spirit and wear the team colors or logo!

33. GIVE THAT PARTY ANIMAL A RIDE

Imagine it's Friday night. Everybody is out and living their best lives. The music is just pumping from the clubs. All the while you are behind the wheel. If you start getting jealous of all the beautiful people, remember why you are there. You're there to pick up the party people that are way too lit and can't take themselves home safely.

Be nice. You might have been in there shoes once before. If you have water or mints, don't hesitate to offer it. You can also bring a barf bag on Fridays and Saturdays driving, you never know when you will truly need it. If accidents happen don't worry, Uber should cover the cleaning costs but will be billed to the rider. The worst part is that you will lose your chance to make some money. Taking your car to detailing can cost you at least a day. Not to mention the lingering barf smell.

34. GIVE SERVICE ANIMALS A LIFT TOO

If you are an animal lover, this may not be a huge hassle for you. But if you aren't one, then you must know that Uber and Lyft require you to accept service animals. Although a former customer told me that he was refused by a prior Uber driver for bringing his dog, it is best to just be prepared instead of risking deactivation. It is required by law for you take service animals, even if you have allergies, a fear of animals, or religious objections.

If you had a dog before, you must also know that some dogs shed more than most. Bringing a lint roller is a good idea to prevent complaints from your next customers. Uber will not compensate you with a cleaning fee. Bring something that can clean doggy spills to prevent complaints from the next rider.

35. PARK IT WHILE IT'S HOT

I initially expected that Uber was going to compensate me for parking fees incurred during rides and deliveries. But as I tried other apps, I realized that none of them do. It is one of the costs that regrettably isn't covered and I frankly find it unfair. Some clients don't even have the common decency to cover your parking costs, so making some deliveries potentially come at a loss.

To prevent additional payments from parking fines, I use the PayBy-Phone app, which is quite useful when you don't have those quarters. I simply place the location code for my car and pay using my debit card. It is especially useful for deliveries since I can extend my time using my phone, when a food pick-up runs longer than I want it to. That means you can put in the minimum amount of time you need and then just extend as needed. It is still best practice to bring quarters just in case.

Postmates used to offers a parking LED that displays their logo and the words "Be right back", so that you can double park, but I doubt it will get you off parking violations. Take my advice and don't risk it. Pay for parking, even if it's just moment. Take the loss.

36. GETTING FOOD ON THE GO

Feeling low? Tired? Bringing a snack can give you that extra push and help you keep focused. When preparing my snack for the road, I keep in mind that it has to not only be energy rich but also handy. One of the easiest snacks to prepare and consume is a hardboiled egg. Just boil them, remove the shell, then pack it. Packing sandwiches is my go-to though, because it can be a complete meal with carbs, fat, and protein. I do this especially when doing deliveries, since that means working when everyone else is eating. It is extra handy when the smell of burgers and fries is making your tummy rumble. Crackers are handy when you are dead hungry and have a passenger. It isn't as intrusive as eating a sandwich or pulling out your hardboiled egg. Just make sure you dust off any food particles from your shirt before handing off your delivery.

37. BRING WATER

It is easy to skip on hydration when you're ridesharing and delivering. After-all you don't want to pee more often than you have to. Taking small frequent sips might help this. Ease up on the coffee as well if you can since it is a diuretic. It will not only make you pee, but also dehydrate you faster.

Use a BPA-free water container for yourself to save on buying water bottles. At the same time, it might be perceived as more sanitary if you use sealed water bottles for your customers. Be careful with leaving water bottles inside your car when it's hot. The heat can melt the plastic and contaminate your water. More research is being conducted for it, but why take the risk?

38. GOING ON A QUEST

If you have played sandbox games like Grand Theft Auto V, then you might be slightly intrigued by doing a Quest with Uber (Boost for Lyft). It's really just a non-gangster version of the pick-up and delivery side-missions in the Grand Theft Auto series. The app felt like my money-making game. It really did remind of playing a videogame since you get a bonus if you complete a certain number of rides at a given time. Just like any videogame, your quest can get more difficult as you progress. The quests can seem unrealistic at times, which will make you wonder if it really is worth it, but it is, what it is.

If you go downtown during rush hour, you can be welcomed with promotions. They're just like quests but it's usually 3 to 5 rides for a bonus, if you stay within the area. Lyft does it different, where your earnings are boosted if you stay in the closest perimeter of a high demand location. Your bonus can increase the longer you are in the perimeter and will hit maximum bonus unless you get a ride notification.

39. KEEP IT HANDY

If you have space to keep in your car, there are some tools that can make your rides safer and ready for simple fixes. Having a tire gauge is an essential tool in your car. Large potholes can offset your tire pressure and can even result in a flat. Saving quarters in the car is useful if you need to inflate your tires at a gas station but it's even handier to have a portable tire-inflator. The one I got can be plugged in your cigarette lighter port. Check your spare monthly to avoid having a useless, deflated spare.

If you owned a crappy old car before, you might have a set of jumper cables handy just in case. But what I learned from the old Ford Contour I used drive, is that you have to have your own battery. My booster is a bit smaller than a car battery and it has cables connected to it. There are smaller ones available now that can be kept in your car just in case.

40. CHECK FOR SPOILS

I'm sure I'm not alone when it comes to leaving things in cab. Thankfully Uber and Lyft make it easier to figure out which car you left your belongings in. Passengers can notify customer service if they left something, then you will be notified of it. You might even get a reward from the person you are returning it to and/or you can even get a "bonus" from Lyft or Uber. Being proactive about it is better. Glancing at the back really quick might get you good tip if you find something. But really, the reward is being able to help someone. Right?

41. KEEP UPDATED

With today's technology, you can get news and updates from everywhere, even from the president. If you have never tried following the twitter of your local traffic news then it would be time to start. Navigation apps can only do so much when it comes to road closures. Keeping updated through twitter and your rideshare apps supplement your map. Being aware of local events that can cause closures or increased traffic can help you plan your day ahead. You prepare yourself on how busy you want to be.

42. GET MATCHING TRIPS

The only thing that makes me feel like I'm actually sharing my ride is being able to match my trips with potential riders. Let's say I had plans to Pike Place Market in Downtown and wasn't in a hurry. Matching my trip would make it more economical since you earn money as you go somewhere. You may have to spend extra time by detouring slightly to pick someone up, but they can also save time by getting you in the carpool lane when the traffic is bad. You get matched to someone that is more or less going towards your direction. Sometimes you can get a matching trip but only have a passenger for a short period of time. You might not even get matched until you get closer to downtown if the demand is low.

Since Uber gives you two matching trips, I save my second matching trip for my way home. If you live by the airport, you may even get more lucrative airport rides.

43. ROADTRIPPING

You might have heard of stories of people booking road trips from LA to Las Vegas. Although I haven't had been hired to drive for four hours, I have actually experienced a trip about for about two hours with a mother and child who just came from the airport.

The first thing you need to do before accepting long trips, is ask yourself if you have the energy to do so. If you end up picking up a passenger with a trip over an hour by mistake and are unable to fulfill the task, politely cancel your trip. If you accepted the trip closer to the time you planned to go home, check your gas tank level. Checking it is crucial if want to decide to power through. If you don't have enough gas, explain to your customer that you will have to stop for gas. If that is acceptable for them, then continue. Try to sneak in some stretching when you help your passengers with the door or with luggage.

44. DOING CAR POOLS

I encountered some challenges when I had my first Uber Pool. My in-app navigation was acting up and didn't have a voice, so I switched to Waze as my default. It became challenging to not be distracted because I had to switch between apps more frequently. Uber Pool or Shared Lyft is when 2 or more users are matched to other users going towards a similar direction. Your pool can end up with different combinations. A mistake I made when I was doing Shared Lyft was me neglecting how many passengers one of the users had. The combination was, one user had two passengers while, the other only had herself. Their pick-up locations were both at the light rail near the university. I accidentally left the user with only one passenger, and just brought the one user with two passengers. I guess until automation happens, they'll have human drivers that make mistakes.

45. MAKE CONVERSATION

Nothing makes a ride feel longer than it should than dead awkward silence. We are social animals. You don't have to have deep meaningful conversation with your passenger but greeting them would be a good start. Be warm and friendly. Smile even through the mirror. If you reflect your guarded nature, then people will be guarded just the same. Talk about the weather if you must. Do what you need to do to make some sort of shallow connection.

46. TALK TO OTHER DRIVERS

The first app that I tried was Uber and it was referred to me. I got a small bonus after, which was nice. When I first started, I thought of the person who referred me as my mentor. I didn't know much about the business except from conversations from other drivers when I was in the Philippines. My conversations with him were useful and it made starting easier. If someone referred you to Uber, maybe talk to them too. Don't be too proud to ask for help. Maybe treat them to coffee as you ask for advice. You can also support bloggers who are spreading information. Buy this book.

47. RATE YOUR RIDERS AND DELIVERIES

Was your customer rude? Condescending? All you have to do is be honest and rate people honestly. I had this useless fear that if I rate any of my passengers low that they would know. Rating is a way to protect yourself as well. If these companies don't know your struggles, then change would not occur. Don't be afraid to hit that 1-star if they really deserve it. Once you fake it and give them more than they deserve, you won't be able to change it. Trust me. I tried going through customer service as petty as it sounded. Sometimes customers have an unattainable expectation with the service you are going to provide them, yet they expect to pay as low as they can. If someone tries to encourage you to do things that can get you in trouble or worse, fined, then politely decline. If they are insistent, try to divert it, then rate them low. You know that they would too.

48. DON'T GET DEACTIVATED

You don't want to stop earning right? There must be some rules that other drivers might have skipped over during signing up, since I see them. I'm never sure if they know it, but you can't have two people operating your Uber. This is a tempting thing to do when you are doing Uber Eats. One person picks up the meals and handles the navigation, and the other just focuses on driving. The money may not be as much after splitting, but it would really make the job easier. Unfortunately, you will have to gamble and risk deactivation when you do this.

Sharing your Uber account is not allowed either. I've had some drivers tell me that they split their car and the account with their significant other, possibly just because it's easier than applying twice. That was even before I started Uber. I called for an Uber and instead of woman driving, I met her husband. It felt sketchy at first, but then he seemed nice and I got where I needed to go. It seems harmless to share your app, but I could have also been a staff for Uber doing quality checks. The app can also catch you by asking you to take a selfie before you can start driving. I'm not a snitch though.

49. YOU GOT TO HUSTLE HARD

Let's be real, you can't really get wealthy from driving for rideshare and delivery apps. I had a stoner smoking in his car, telling me to get a real job. Some days it can get really low. You have to break more than a sweat to stay profitable. You have to scramble to get gigs, switching from app to app. You just have to keep cool and continue plugging. A consistent common denominator to these apps is that it won't be a permanent thing. They don't want permanent workers. They want you to come and go as you please. They want your earnings to be inconsistent. Just try to remember why you started the hustle. Remember that goal, hit it, and move forward. Maybe even expand your goals and business. Think bigger. It is not too late as long as you are living. Maybe after learning all you can about Uber, you can start a fleet of Ubers. You can even write a book or start a Youtube channel about it. Do not limit the hustle.

50. BE FUN! HAVE FUN!

What's the point of owning your own business if you can't enjoy it? Owning your business can have its own stress, and some days you will ask yourself if you should have stayed as an employee. The odds can be staggering after all. Keeping your head up is all you can do some days. It's the positive thing to do anyway. Visualize the day you hit your long-term goals. Think about how you can hit your short-term goals. Enjoy yourself because you are on your way. Make it show when you drive. Let your customers know that you appreciate their business. Take care of your customers food like it's your food. The importance you show in your job will reflect on others. Keep your work ethics, even when it's tempting to just take shortcuts. No job is too small. Continue to be generous, even when customers aren't. Appreciate the time you give to this. You're not on your couch dreaming of how to get rich. You are moving. Doing something. Have fun chief.

OTHER HELPFUL RESOURCES

57 Million Workers are Part of the Gig Economy - https://www.forbes.com/sites/tjmccue/2018/08/31/57-million-u-s-workers-are-part-of-the-gig-economy/#7207e7f57118

What is a Gig Worker? - https://www.gigeconomydata.org/basics/what-gig-worker

History of Uber - https://www.uber.com/newsroom/history/

Uber Payments - https://www.uber.com/en-GH/drive/resources/payments/

Lyft Files For IPO - https://www.latimes.com/business/la-fi-lyft-ipo-uber-20190301-story.html

Uber Fees - https://www.ridester.com/uber-fees/

Square Acquires Caviar - https://techcrunch.com/2014/08/04/its-official-square-acquires-food-delivery-service-caviar/

About Square - https://squareup.com/us/en/about

TNC Permit - http://www.seattle.gov/business-regulations/taxis-for-hires-and-tncs/transportation-network-companies

TNC - http://www.seattle.gov/business-regulations/taxis-for-hires-and-tncs/transportation-network-companies/tnc-drivers

Go Bank - https://www.businesswire.com/news/home/20160317005466/en/Green-Dot-Uber-Announce-Uber-Checking-GoBank%C2%AE

Stash - https://www.stashinvest.com/invest

Brownbear - https://www.brownbear.com/why-us/wash-green

Holding Pee - https://www.healthline.com/health/holding-pee

Bladder Raptures - https://health.howstuffworks.com/human-body/systems/kidney-urinary/hold-pee-so-long-bladder-ruptures.htm

Uber and Service Animals - https://www.latimes.com/business/technology/la-fi-tn-uber-service-animals-20160715-snap-story.html

Service Animal Policy - https://accessibility.uber.com/service-animal-policy/

Don't Drink that Bottled Water - https://www.thoughtco.com/viral-warning-dont-drink-bottled-water-left-in-car-3299593

READ OTHER 50 THINGS TO KNOW BOOKS

50 Things to Know to Get Things Done Fast: Easy Tips for Success

50 Things to Know About Going Green: Simple Changes to Start Today

50 Things to Know to Live a Happy Life Series

50 Things to Know to Organize Your Life: A Quick Start Guide to Declutter, Organize, and Live Simply

50 Things to Know About Being a Minimalist: Downsize, Organize, and Live Your Life

50 Things to Know About Speed Cleaning: How to Tidy Your Home in Minutes

50 Things to Know About Choosing the Right Path in Life

50 Things to Know to Get Rid of Clutter in Your Life: Evaluate, Purge, and Enjoy Living

50 Things to Know About Journal Writing: Exploring Your Innermost Thoughts & Feelings

READ OTHER 50 THINGS TO KNOW BOOKS

50 Things to Know to Get Things Done Fast: Easy Tips for Success

50 Things to Know About Going Green: Simple Changes to Start Today

50 Things to Know to Live a Happy Life Series

50 Things to Know to Organize Your Life: A Quick Start Guide to Declutter, Organize, and Live Simply

50 Things to Know About Being a Minimalist: Downsize, Organize, and Live Your Life

50 Things to Know About Speed Cleaning: How to Tidy Your Home in Minutes

50 Things to Know About Choosing the Right Path in Life

50 Things to Know to Get Rid of Clutter in Your Life: Evaluate, Purge, and Enjoy Living

50 Things to Know About Journal Writing: Exploring Your Innermost Thoughts & Feelings

50 Things to Know

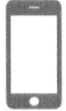

Website: 50thingstoknow.com

Facebook: facebook.com/50thingstoknow

Pinterest: pinterest.com/lbrennec

YouTube: youtube.com/user/50ThingsToKnow

Twitter: twitter.com/50ttk

Mailing List: Join the 50 Things to Know Mailing List to Learn About New Releases

50 Things to Know

Please leave your honest review of this book on Amazon and Goodreads. We appreciate your positive and constructive feedback. Thank you.

www.ingramcontent.com/pod-product-compliance
Lightning Source LLC
Chambersburg PA
CBHW030728180526
45157CB00008BA/3093